God's greatest desire is for us to live victorious lives and continually enjoy his blessings bequeathed to us. As God is Spirit & Man also is a Spirit so Walk in divine excellence and transform your world through the power of a renewed mind.

Topic

Symbol	Disease, Symptoms, Risk factor & Remedy
A	Rheumatoid arthritis
B	Homeopathic treatment of RA
C	Most effective Remedy
D	Osteoarthritis (OA)
E	Homeopathic treatment of OA
F	Most effective Remedy
G	Ayurveda in Rheumatoid arthritis
H	Ayurveda in Osteoarthritis arthritis

Rheumatoid arthritis (RA)

1. What is Rheumatoid arthritis (RA)

- Rheumatoid arthritis (RA) is an autoimmune disease in which the body's immune system – which normally protects its health by attacking foreign substances like bacteria and viruses – mistakenly attacks the joints. This creates inflammation that causes the tissue that lines the inside of joints (the synovium) to thicken, resulting in swelling and pain in and around the joints. The synovium makes a fluid that lubricates joints and helps them move smoothly.

- Rheumatoid arthritis most commonly affects the joints of the hands, feet, wrists, elbows, knees and ankles. The joint effect is usually symmetrical. That means if one knee or hand if affected, usually the other one is, too. Because RA also can affect body systems, such as the cardiovascular or respiratory systems, it is called a systemic disease. Systemic means "entire body."

2. Who is Affected by Rheumatoid Arthritis?

- In women, RA most commonly begins between ages 30 and 60.

- In men, it often occurs later in life.

- Having a family member with RA increases the odds of having RA; however, the majority of people with RA have no family history of the disease.

- Teenagers also may suffer.

3. Rheumatoid Arthritis Causes

- An abnormal response of the immune system plays a leading role in the inflammation and joint damage that occurs. No one knows for sure why the immune system goes awry, but there is scientific evidence that genes, hormones and environmental factors are involved.

- Researchers have shown that people with a specific genetic marker called the HLA shared epitope have a fivefold greater chance of developing rheumatoid arthritis than do people without the marker. The HLA genetic site controls immune responses. Other genes connected to RA include: STAT4, a gene that plays important roles in the regulation and activation of the immune system; TRAF1 and C5, two genes relevant to chronic inflammation; and PTPN22, a gene associated with both the development and progression of rheumatoid arthritis. Yet not all people with these genes develop RA and not all people with the condition have these genes.

- Researchers continue to investigate other factors that may play a role. These factors include infectious agents such as bacteria or viruses, which may trigger development of the disease in a person whose genes make them more likely to get it; female hormones (70 percent of people with RA are women); obesity; and the body's response to stressful events such as physical or emotional trauma.

- Research also has indicated that environmental factors may play a role in one's risk for rheumatoid arthritis. Some include exposure to cigarette smoke, air pollution, insecticides and occupational exposures to mineral oil and silica.

4. Rheumatoid Arthritis Symptoms

1. In the early stages, people with RA may not initially see redness or swelling in the joints, but they may experience tenderness and pain.

2. These following joint symptoms are clues to RA:

- Joint pain, tenderness, swelling or stiffness for six weeks or longer
- Morning stiffness for 30 minutes or longer
- More than one joint is affected
- Small joints (wrists, certain joints of the hands and feet) are affected
- The same joints on both sides of the body are affected

3. Along with pain, many people experience fatigue, loss of appetite and a low-grade fever.

4. The symptoms and effects of RA may come and go. A period of high disease activity (increases in inflammation and other symptoms) is called a flare. A flare can last for days or months.

5. Homeopathic treatment (Natural Cure)

- Causticum 30,
- Dulcamara 30,
- Rhododendron chrysanthum 30,
- Rhus toxicodendron 30
- Nux vomica 30,
- Berberis vulgaris 30,
- Calcarea phosphorica 30,

6. Most effective Remedy

- Dr. Reckeweg R-11, Homeopathic Medicine (15 drops in 1/2 cup of water 3 or 4 times a day)

    "For complete healing "Continue above medicine for one or two years"

Osteoarthritis (OA)

7. What is Osteoarthritis?

- Sometimes called degenerative joint disease or degenerative arthritis, osteoarthritis (OA) is the most common chronic condition of the joints, affecting approximately 27 million Americans.

- OA can affect any joint, but it occurs most often in knees, hips, lower back and neck, small joints of the fingers and the bases of the thumb and big toe.

- In normal joints, a firm, rubbery material called cartilage covers the end of each bone. Cartilage provides a smooth, gliding surface for joint motion and acts as a cushion between the bones. In OA, the cartilage breaks down, causing pain, swelling and problems moving the joint.

- As OA worsens over time, bones may break down and develop growths called spurs. Bits of bone or cartilage may chip off and float around in the joint.

- In the body, an inflammatory process occurs and cytokines (proteins) and enzymes develop that further damage the cartilage. In the final stages of OA, the cartilage wears away and bone rubs against bone leading to joint damage and more pain.

Who's Affected?

Although OA occurs in people of all ages, osteoarthritis is most common in people older than 65. Common risk factors include increasing age, obesity, previous joint injury, overuse of the joint, weak thigh muscles, and genes.

- One in two adults will develop symptoms of knee OA during their lives.
- One in four adults will develop symptoms of hip OA by age 85.
- One in 12 people 60 years or older have hand OA.

8. Osteoarthritis Symptoms

Symptoms of osteoarthritis vary, depending on which joints are affected and how severely they are affected. However, the most common symptoms are pain and stiffness, particularly first thing in the morning or after resting. Affected joints may get swollen, especially after extended activity. These symptoms tend to build over time rather than show

up suddenly. Some of the common symptoms include:

Sore or stiff joints – particularly the hips, knees, and lower back – after inactivity or overuse.

- Limited range of motion or stiffness that goes away after movement
- Clicking or cracking sound when a joint bends
- Mild swelling around a joint
- Pain that is worse after activity or toward the end of the day

Here are ways OA may affect different parts of the body:

- Hips. Pain is felt in the groin area or buttocks and sometimes on the inside of the knee or thigh.
- Knees. A "grating" or "scraping" sensation occurs when moving the knee.
- Fingers. Bony growths (spurs) at the edge of joints can cause fingers to become swollen, tender and red. There may be pain at the base of the thumb.

- Feet. Pain and tenderness is felt in the large joint at the base of the big toe. There may be swelling in ankles or toes.

- OA pain, swelling or stiffness may make it difficult to perform ordinary tasks at work or at home. Simple acts like tucking in bed sheets, opening a box of food, grasping a computer mouse or driving a car can become nearly impossible. When the lower body joints are affected, activities such as walking, climbing stairs and lifting objects may become difficult. When finger and hand joints are affected, osteoarthritis can make it difficult to grasp and hold objects, such as a pencil, or to do delicate tasks, such as needlework.

Many people believe that the effects of osteoarthritis are inevitable, so they don't do anything to manage it. OA symptoms can hinder work, social life and family life if steps are not taken to prevent joint damage, manage pain and increase flexibility.

How OA May Affect Overall Health

- The pain, reduced mobility, side effects from medication and other factors associated with osteoarthritis can lead to negative health effects not directly related to the joint disease.

Diabetes and Heart Disease

- Knee or hip pain may lead to a sedentary lifestyle that promotes weight gain and possible obesity. Being overweight or obese can lead to the development of diabetes, heart disease and high blood pressure.

Falls

- People with osteoarthritis experience as much as 30 percent more falls and have a 20 percent greater risk of fracture than those without OA. People with OA have risk factors such as decreased function, muscle weakness and impaired balance that make them more likely to fall. Side effects from medications used for pain relief can also contribute to falls. Narcotic pain relievers can cause people to feel dizzy and unbalanced.

9. Osteoarthritis Causes

Although osteoarthritis was long believed to be caused by the "wear and tear" of joints over time, scientists now view it as a disease of the joint. Here are some of the factors that contribute to the development of OA:

Genes:

- Various genetic traits can make a person more likely to develop OA. One possibility is a rare defect in the body's production of collagen, the protein that makes up cartilage. This abnormality can cause osteoarthritis to occur as early as age 20. Other inherited traits may result in slight defects in the way the bones fit together so that cartilage wears away faster than usual. Researchers have found that a gene called FAAH, previously linked to increased pain sensitivity, is higher in people with knee OA than in people who don't have the disease.

Weight:

- Being overweight puts additional pressure on hips and knees. Many years of carrying extra pounds can cause the cartilage that cushions joints to break down faster. Research has shown there is a link between being overweight and having an increased risk of osteoarthritis in the hands. These studies suggest that excess fat tissue produces inflammatory chemicals (cytokines) that can damage the joints.

Injury and overuse:

- Repetitive movements or injuries to joints (such as a fracture, surgery or ligament tears) can lead to osteoarthritis. Some athletes, for example, repeatedly damage joints, tendons and ligaments, which can speed cartilage breakdown. Certain careers that require standing for long periods of time, repetitive bending, heavy lifting or other movements can also make cartilage wear away more quickly. An imbalance or weakness of the muscles supporting a joint can also lead to altered movement and eventual cartilage breakdown in joints.

Others:

- Several other factors may contribute to osteoarthritis. These factors include bone and joint disorders like rheumatoid arthritis, certain metabolic disorders such as hemochromatosis, which causes the body to absorb too much iron, or acromegaly, which causes the body to make too much growth hormone.

10. Osteoarthritis Diagnosis

To diagnose osteoarthritis, the doctor will collect information on personal and family medical history, perform a physical examination and order diagnostic tests.

Health History and Symptoms

The information needed to help diagnose osteoarthritis includes:

- Description of the symptoms
- Details about when and how the pain or other symptoms began

- Details about other medical problems that exist
- Location of the pain, stiffness or other symptoms
- How the symptoms affect daily activities
- List of current medications

Physical Examination

- During the exam, the doctor will examine the joints and test their range of motion (how well each joint moves through its full range). He will be looking for areas that are tender, painful or swollen as well as signs of joint damage. The doctor will examine the position and alignment of the neck and spine.

Diagnostic Tests

A diagnosis of osteoarthritis may be suspected after a medical history and physical examination is done. Blood tests are usually not helpful in making a diagnosis. However, the following tests may help confirm it:

- **Joint aspiration.**

    The doctor will numb the affected area and insert a needle into the joint to withdraw fluid. The fluid will be examined for evidence of crystals or joint deterioration. This test can help rule out other medical conditions or other forms of arthritis.

- **X-ray.**

X-rays can show damage and other changes related to osteoarthritis to confirm the diagnosis.

- **MRI.**

    Magnetic resonance imaging (MRI) does not use radiation. It is more expensive than X-rays, but will provide a view that offers better images of cartilage and other structures to detect early abnormalities typical of osteoarthritis.

> 11. Osteoarthritis Prevention: What You Can Do

Osteoarthritis does not have to be a foregone conclusion as you age. Find out what you can do to stave off OA.

- (OA) was once considered a disorder in which joints simply wore out – the unavoidable result of a long and active life.

- But research has shown that OA is a complex process with many causes. It is not an inevitable part of aging experts say, but rather the result of a combination of factors, many of which can be modified or prevented.

Here is what doctors recommend to reduce the risk of OA or delay its onset.

Maintain a Healthy Weight

Excess weight is one of the biggest risk factors for osteoarthritis – and for good reason. Extra pounds put additional pressure on weight-bearing joints, such as the hips and knees. Each pound you gain adds nearly four pounds of stress to your knees and increases pressure on your hips six-fold. Over time, the extra strain breaks down the cartilage that cushions these joints.

But mechanical stress is not the only problem. Fat tissue produces proteins called cytokines that promote inflammation throughout the body. In the joints, cytokines destroy tissue by altering the function of cartilage cells. When you gain weight, your body makes and releases more of these destructive proteins. Unless you are very overweight, losing even a few pounds can reduce joint stress and inflammation, cutting your risk of OA in half.

Control Blood Sugar

The latest research suggests that diabetes, which affects the body's ability to regulate blood sugar (glucose), may be a significant risk factor for osteoarthritis. That's because high glucose levels speed the formation of certain molecules that make cartilage stiffer and more sensitive to mechanical stress. Diabetes can also trigger systemic inflammation that leads to cartilage loss. The newly discovered connection between diabetes and joint damage may help explain why more than half of Americans diagnosed with diabetes also have arthritis.

Get Physical

Physical activity is the best available treatment for OA. It's also one of the best ways to keep joints healthy in the first place. As little as 30 minutes of moderately intense exercise five times a week helps joints stay limber and strengthens the muscles that support and stabilize your hips and knees. Exercise also strengthens the heart and lungs, lowers diabetes risk and is a key factor in weight control.

You don't have to join a gym or have a formal workout plan to benefit. Walking, gardening – even scrubbing floors – count. But the greatest results come with a consistent and progressive exercise program adjusted for your age, fitness level and the activities you enjoy most.

No matter what type of exercise you choose, listen to your body. If you have pain after a workout that persists more than an hour or two, do less next time and take more breaks. To avoid injury, go slow until you know how your body reacts to a new activity and don't repeat the same exercise every day. If you have a hard time starting or sticking with an exercise program, the Arthritis Foundation's Walk With Ease program can help you reach your goals.

Play it Safe

Because cartilage doesn't heal well, an injured joint is nearly seven times more likely to develop arthritis than one that was never injured. Fractures, dislocations – even ligament tears and strains – can significantly increase the risk of OA, which occurs in about 50 percent of people who experience a traumatic injury.

Although injuries aren't always avoidable, it pays to protect your joints. If you play sports, wear protective gear, such as joint padding for soccer or hockey. And make sure any baseball field you use has break-away bases. At home or work, use your largest, strongest joints for lifting and carrying and take breaks when you need to. After an injury, maintaining a healthy weight can help guard against further joint damage.

Choose a Healthy Lifestyle

Some risk factors for OA can't be changed. For instance, OA becomes more common as people age, though why this occurs isn't clear. One idea is that the number of cartilage cells simply diminishes over time. Because more women than men develop OA, especially after age 50, lower estrogen levels after menopause may also play a role.

In addition, some people inherit genes that make them more susceptible to OA. In one study, variations in the gene for a cytokine associated with inflammation and cartilage loss doubled the risk of severe arthritis. It's important to remember, though, that arthritis is a multi factorial disorder and simply inheriting a gene doesn't mean you will develop it.

Ultimately, the best defense against any disease, including OA, is a healthy lifestyle. The way you eat, exercise, sleep, manage stress and interact with others, and whether you smoke or drink can have a tremendous influence not just on overall health, but also on the health of your joints.

12 . Homeopathic treatment   (Natural Cure)

- Rhus toxicidendron 30,
- Bryonia alba 30,

- Arnica Montana 30,
- Calcaria fluoride 30,
- Calcaria carbonate 30,
- Pulsatilla nigra 30,
- Radium bromide 30,
- Kali carbonicum 30, etc

Best Remedy

- Dr. Reckeweg R-73, Homeopathic Medicine (15 drops in 1/2 cup of water 3 or 4 times a day)

Active ingredients

- Arnica montana, radix 4X 2 g,
- Bryonia 4X 2 g,
- Ledum palustre 4X 2 g,
- Sulphuricum acidum 6X 2 g,
- Argentum metallicum 12X 1 g,
- Causticum 12X 1 g in 10 g.

> 13. Ayurveda about Rheumatoid arthritis (RA)

Ayurveda is an traditional Indian practice involving a natural, holistic approach to treating medical conditions.

Some Ayurvedic practitioners use Ayurveda to treat rheumatoid arthritis (RA), which they call "amavata." Ayurvedic treatment can include supplements, dietary changes, and exercise.

This article will review Ayurvedic treatment for RA, including the basic principles and whether research supports its use.

14. General principles

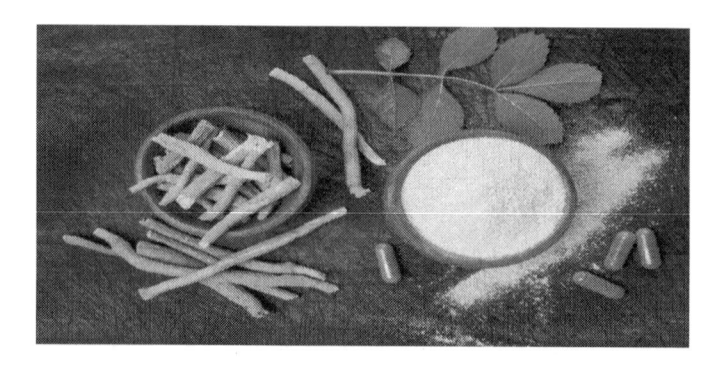

Ayurvedic treatments often involve herbal remedies, such as ashwagandha.

The term "Ayurveda" is a combination of two Sanskrit terms "ayu" (life) and "veda" (knowledge). Practitioners work to balance the three energy forces, or "doshas," of life: "vata," "pitta," and "kapha."

Ayurvedic treatments for RA depend on which diagnostic guidelines the practitioner uses.

For example, those who practice from the guidelines "Madhava Nidana" believe that imbalances in the gut and inflammatory compounds cause RA.

On the other hand, practitioners from the "Ashtanga Hridaya" school of thought believe that RA is the result of poor dietary and lifestyle habits that cause inflammation in the body.

Both approaches use herbs, supplements, dietary changes, and exercise to help relieve RA symptoms.

15. Herbs and supplements

Ayurvedic practice often involves the use of herbs and supplements as treatment.

Some of the herbs that Ayurvedic practitioners often use to treat RA include:

- *Boswellia serrata* (Indian frankincense)
- garlic
- ginger
- *Ricinus communis* (castor oil)
- ashwagandha

Some Ayurvedic medicine formulations also contain "bhasma," which are specially prepared forms of metals, such as silver, copper, and iron.

An Ayurvedic practitioner may also prepare special oils that contain herbs. People can massage these oils into areas where they experience symptoms.

The Food and Drug Administration (FDA) do not regulate Ayurvedic supplements in the same way as prescription medications.

As a result, less information is available about how supplements work, how they may interact with other prescription medications, and if they are safe.

For this reason, it is vital that people only purchase Ayurvedic supplements from a reputable practitioner and tell their doctor if they are using Ayurvedic treatments.

They should also ask their Ayurvedic practitioner exactly what is in each preparation to ensure that it does not contain compounds that a person is allergic to or that may interact with other medical treatments.

16. Diet

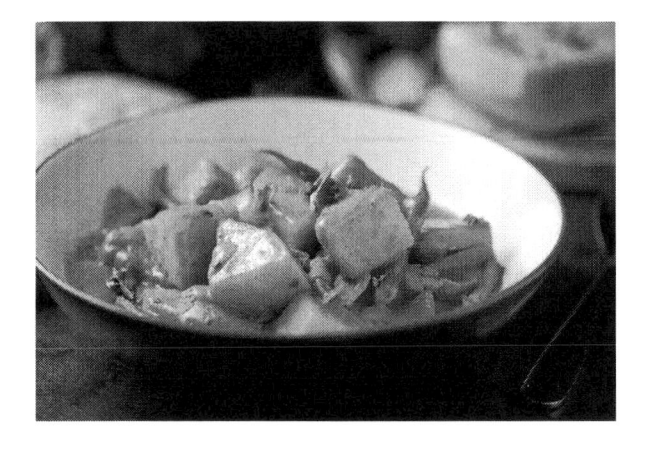

According to Ayurveda, certain foods may worsen RA symptoms.

Ayurvedic practitioners believe the following dietary habits may cause or worsen the symptoms of RA:

- drinking alcohol
- eating spicy foods
- taking in excess salt
- consuming too many sour, sweet, or sugary foods
- eating uncooked foods
- eating foods that cause **acid reflux**

As a result, an Ayurvedic practitioner will recommend avoiding these foods.

Some Ayurvedic practitioners also recommend soups that contain barley and rice, as these are thought to add a sense of lightness to the body.

Sometimes, a practitioner may recommend a castor oil fast. This is when a person consumes castor oil, a natural laxative, to encourage intestinal purification.

Over several days, a person will reintroduce foods and ultimately progress to a healthful routine diet.

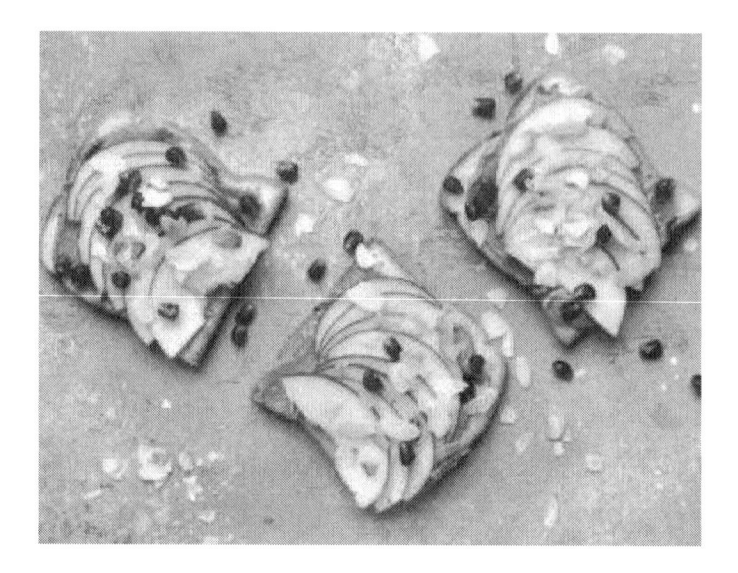

What can you eat on an anti-inflammatory diet?

An anti-inflammatory diet is another holistic approach to treating rheumatoid arthritis. Learn more about it here.

Exercise and lifestyle

Ayurvedic practitioners believe that positive lifestyle habits can support RA treatment.

They believe that a sedentary lifestyle leads to the formation of "ama," which causes inflammation and disease.

Practicing yoga, an essential part of Ayurvedic medicine, can help a person with RA to be more active and also reduce stiffness and pain.

Ayurvedic practitioners may recommend the following tips for people with RA:

- using hot water, not cold, to bathe in and drink
- avoiding exposure to cold breezes
- avoiding late-night or late-afternoon naps
- practicing yoga to relieve mental stress
- using massage therapy with herbal oils to reduce pain and stiffness

While Ayurvedic practitioners do believe that physical activity can help relieve some conditions, they recommend that people with RA avoid excess walking.

What does the research say?

Little extensive and modern research exists on Ayurvedic treatments specifically for RA.

Researchers report difficulties designing clinical trials to test Ayurvedic interventions, compared with modern medicine or **placebos**. Many studies are small, making it difficult for researchers to know if the results would apply to larger populations.

For example, a 2011 study published in the *International Journal of Ayurveda Research* studied Ayurvedic treatments in 290 people with RA over 7 years.

At the study's conclusion, the author found that even participants with severe RA reported improvements, including reductions in swelling and pain. However, the study did not use a control group, so the conclusions are difficult to confirm.

Other, smaller case studies support the use of Ayurveda in treating individuals with RA.

A **2015 case report** on Ayurvedic treatment in a 45-year-old female supported the use of Ayurveda for reducing RA symptoms. The treatment included massage, supplements, a castor oil fast, avoiding spicy foods, and eating "light" foods.

Some aspects of Ayurvedic treatment have more support in contemporary research. For example, many Ayurvedic practitioners recommend yoga to help relieve RA symptoms.

A **2018 study** on 75 adults with RA found that yoga improved fitness, flexibility, mood, and overall health-related quality of life.

Summary

Unfortunately, little high-quality research exists to support the use of Ayurvedic treatments for RA.

However, with a doctor's supervision, many of the dietary and exercise-related changes may be beneficial. Also, any reduction in inflammation is likely beneficial. Since RA can damage joints without effective treatment, working with a rheumatology doctor along with an Ayurvedic practitioner is important.

Currently, there is no licensing program for Ayurvedic practitioners in the United States, nor is there an official training or certification process. This is different from Ayurvedic training in India, which has many regulations.

Anyone considering Ayurvedic treatment should speak to their regular doctor and be sure to ask about an Ayurvedic practitioner's training and safety practices.

An Ayurvedic Approach to Osteoarthritis

Osteoarthritis (OA) is a chronic condition of the joints in which the cartilage cushioning the ends of the bones gradually loses its elasticity and wears away. Without the protective cartilage, the bones begin to rub against each other, causing stiffness, inflammation, and loss of movement. Osteoarthritis treatment therapies with current conventional medicine typically focuses on pain reduction and control of inflammation; however, these approaches have no effect on the natural course of the disease.

The most common medications prescribed for osteoarthritis are, at best, moderately effective. In addition, side effects of these treatments can be quite significant, and at times life-threatening. Often times, the ultimate treatment for a disabling joint is joint replacement, with the inherent risks and cost that come with surgery. If current trends continue, it is estimated that 600,000 hip replacements and 1.4 million knee replacements will be carried out in the U.S. alone in 2015.

Osteoarthritis is the most common form of arthritis worldwide, with symptoms ranging from minor discomfort to debilitation. It can occur in any of the body's joints but most often develops in the hands and weight-bearing joints, including the knees, hips, and spine (usually in the neck or lower back). For people coping with advanced osteoarthritis, the effects are not only physical but also emotional as pain and decreasing mobility can limit the ability to work, participate in daily activities with friends and family, and enjoy life.

What Causes Osteoarthritis?

While science has no definite answers about what causes OA, researchers have identified several factors involved in the development and course of OA. Some of these factors include inflammation, biomechanical imbalances that put stress on the joints, and cellular disorders that lead to the abnormal breakdown of cartilage. It is important that the approach we use in treating OA address as many of these factors as possible.

Ayurvedic Approaches to Osteoarthritis

Given the only moderate effectiveness and potential side effects of conventional treatment, both patients and health care professionals are seeking out alternative therapies, including those offered by the ancient healing system known as Ayurveda. In this article we'll look at the three main modalities Ayurveda uses to treat osteoarthritis and other disorders: herbal treatments, meditation, and yoga.

Ayurvedic Herbal Treatments

Ayurveda offers many herbal treatments for the treatment of OA. These plants have documented anti-inflammatory properties without the side effects of commonly prescribed medications. For example, at a recent meeting of the American College of Rheumatology, a study was presented that showed an herbal Ayurvedic therapy to be as effective in treating knee osteoarthritis as a commonly prescribed medication (Celebrex) and glucosamine – and with fewer side effects. The ACR stated that

Ayurveda offers "safe and effective treatment alternatives" for OA.

The herbs boswellia, turmeric, ashwagandha, ginger, triphala, guggulu, and shatavari have all been shown to decrease inflammation by interfering with the production of inflammatory chemicals in the body.

Boswellia

There is evidence that the Ayurvedic herb Boswellia serrata, also called Indian frankincense, alleviates joint pain and inflammation. Boswellia blocks an enzyme (5-lipoxygenase) that plays a major role in the formation of chemicals called leukotrienes, which stimulate and perpetuate inflammation. Researchers have found that people with osteoarthritis who took boswellia along with ashwagandha, turmeric, and zinc reported less joint pain and increased mobility and strength.

Turmeric

Turmeric is a spice commonly used in South and East Asian cooking. It is also used both orally and topically in traditional

Ayurvedic medicine to treat a wide variety of ailments, many of which are related to inflammation. The active ingredient in turmeric, curcumin, has been shown to inhibit key inflammation-producing enzymes (lipo-oxygenase, cyclo-oxygenase, and phospholipase A2), thus disrupting the inflammatory cascade at three different stages. Interestingly, some data suggests that it may protect the stomach against non-steroidal anti-inflammatories (NSAIDs). Although current studies for its use in treating osteoarthritis are few, curcumin/turmeric is a promising option in the treatment of OA.

Ashwagandha

Another Ayurvedic herb, ashwagandha (Withania somnifera), has known anti-inflammatory effects. In a study published in 2007, the extract of this herb was found to suppress the production of pro-inflammatory molecules (TNF-alpha and two interleukin subtypes. In one study, the anti-inflammatory effect of ashwagandha was comparable to taking the steroid hydrocortisone.

Ginger

The anti-inflammatory effects of ginger (Zinziber officinale) have also been documented. Ginger works as an anti-inflammatory by interfering with an enzyme (cyclooxygenase) that produces inflammatory chemicals in the body. There is some data showing that ginger has a moderate beneficial effect on OA of the knee. Further research is needed to determine the extent of ginger's effectiveness in treating OA.

Triphala

The Ayurvedic herb triphala has been used in India for thousands of years for treatment of osteoarthritis. Triphala is a formulary that consists of three herbs (amalaki, haritaki, and bibhitaki). Preliminary studies show that the herbs in triphala have anti-inflammatory effects.

Guggulu

In addition, the herb guggulu (Commiphora guggul) has been shown to be a potent inhibitor of the enzyme NFKB, which regulates the body's inflammatory response. There are several studies that show decreased inflammation and joint swelling after administration of extracts of guggulu resin.

Shatavari

Shatavari (Asparagus racemosus) is an Ayurvedic herb that is considered to have a soothing, cooling, and lubricating influence on the body. Studies have found that it has an inhibitory effect on chemicals that create inflammation in the body, such as TNF-alpha, and IL-1B.

The Benefits of Meditation

An important principle in Ayurveda is acknowledgment of the importance of the emotional and spiritual aspects of health and healing. Health is achieved by balancing not only the body, but mind and spirit as well. Meditation provides a way to achieve this balance. The practice of meditation also creates many physiological changes, including reduction of inflammation in the body.

Mind-body practices such as meditation have value as part of a treatment regimen for chronic pain caused by a variety of conditions.

Although to date there are no studies specifically done on the effects of meditation on osteoarthritis, several studies have shown that mindfulness meditation can be useful in the treatment of pain syndromes.

A landmark study conducted in 1982 showing the beneficial effect of meditation on pain reduction was carried out by Dr. Jon Kabat-Zinn with a group of patients suffering from chronic pain. After completing a ten-week program of mindfulness meditation, 65 percent of the participants showed a significant reduction in pain levels. Since then, many other studies have confirmed these findings.

A Tool to Diminish Feelings of Pain

Researchers have found that through the regular practice of meditation, we can actually change how our mind perceives pain. Meditation doesn't take the sensation of pain away; it develops our capacity for detached observation, which helps us separate our experience of physical sensations from the painful stories and emotions we generate in reaction to those sensations.

Emotional reactions such as anxiety, fear, and depression intensify feelings of pain. As many studies have found, meditation is a powerful tool for training our minds to regulate our emotions, reduce anticipation of pain, and increase relaxation – thereby decreasing our perception of pain.

Meditation Enhances Conventional Treatment

Another notable study by Randolph in 1999 found that meditation in conjunction with conventional medical treatment medicine enhances the effectiveness of Western medical treatment alone. In this study, patients were taught hatha yoga and meditation in two-hour classes.

A year later, patients undergoing the pain and stress management program in addition to the medical treatment reported that their feelings of pain decreased by 79 percent.

Meditation is an important healing tool that uses the mind-body connection to help people deal with pain conditions, such as OA. Meditation is fast becoming recognized as an effective way of reducing pain. The American Pain Foundation

acknowledges the use of meditation and offers many resources for meditation. By using meditation as part of a comprehensive treatment regimen for OA, patients have the potential to experience less pain and suffering.

By addressing pain in a holistic sense, instead of just as a physical problem, meditation offers the opportunity to use the mind to influence the experience of pain.

Releasing the Stress of Chronic Pain

In addition to the emotional regulation of pain, meditation can help deal with the stress associated with living with a chronic pain condition. Since the 1960s, numerous studies have been done on the physiologic effects of meditation. These studies show that meditation results in the opposite of the physiological changes that occur during the stress response. When we're faced with stress, whether physical or emotional, our body reacts with the fight-or-flight response: our heart beats faster, our blood pressure rises, our breath becomes shallow, our adrenalin and cortisol production surge, our blood sugar rises, we produce lower levels of sex hormones, and our immune system weakens.

In contrast, during meditation, our body enters a state of restful awareness. When we have a regular meditation practice, the physical and emotional healing benefits include:

- Decreased blood pressure and hypertension
- Slower heart rate
- Lower cholesterol levels
- Reduced production of "stress hormones," including cortisol and adrenaline
- More efficient oxygen use by the body
- Increased production of the anti-aging hormone DHEA
- Improved immune function and more restful sleep

Getting Started with Meditation

There is an enormous variety of meditation techniques available, and it's important to find one that resonates with you. The Chopra Center offers instruction in an easy-to-learn practice called Primordial Sound Meditation. Many people have also benefitted from using guided meditations and visualizations.

Yoga for Osteoarthritis

Yoga is a time-honored science for balanced living and self-realization. By integrating body, mind, and spirit with the practice of yoga, we experience physical, emotional and spiritual benefits. In addition, by bringing our attention to the present moment, we increase our body awareness, not only while practicing yoga, but also in our everyday movements.

From a physical perspective, the practice of yoga increases strength, flexibility, and balance, all of which are important for health in general and are particularly vital for those coping with osteoarthritis (OA).

When practiced regularly, gentle yoga movements not only strengthen the muscles that support the joints but also improve the flexibility of the muscles, which is more effective than just strengthening alone. Several studies have shown the benefit of stretching and increasing flexibility for people with OA in the knees.

While some exercise programs focus solely on strengthening the quadriceps muscle (an important part of most approaches to knee OA), including yoga stretches builds strength as well as increasing flexibility. One study that focused exclusively on quadriceps strengthening demonstrated that patients actually lost flexibility when they only focused on strength training. This did not occur in programs that included stretching.

Relieving Stress on the Joints

Yoga's focus on balance and alignment helps improve biomechanical imbalances that create stress on the joints. As researchers have found, the damage to cartilage often occurs because of the unbalanced positions that the body is put in while sitting, walking, and moving. Misalignments of bones, dysfunctional movement patterns, lack of body awareness, and poor posture can all contribute to wear and tear of the cartilage. Yoga can retrain our body to move in ways that decrease stress on our joints.

Moving

Another benefit of yoga is that it keeps people moving and reduces the pain and stiffness associated with osteoarthritis. Over time, lack of movement leads to tighter muscles and lack of circulation into the joints themselves. Movement is necessary for proper production of the synovial fluid inside the joints. By moving the joints, the synovial fluid can continuously lubricate and cushion the joints.

People with "loose" or hyper mobile joints have a higher risk of developing OA due to uneven wear and tear on the joints. In this case, yoga can be used as a therapy to stabilize hyper mobile joints by strengthening the muscles around joints and eliminating the uneven forces on the joint.

Yoga Enhances Emotional Wellbeing

Beyond the physical improvements that yoga can provide, it has the additional benefits of enhancing mental well-being and emotional balance. Yoga is associated with increased energy, fewer bodily aches and pains, and increased mental energy and positive feelings. These are all important factors for anyone dealing with chronic pain conditions such as OA.

How to Get Started with Yoga

If you're using yoga as a therapeutic tool for OA and other conditions, it's important to work with a certified yoga instructor or therapist to develop a specific program that is appropriate for your individual needs. Here I will offer some general guidance and descriptions of a few poses that target specific areas of the body.

- Always listen to your body and never go beyond what is comfortable.

- Yoga is not a competitive sport; every body is different, so don't compare your yoga practice with anyone else's.
- Focus on the breath with each pose to connect you to the present moment
- All poses can be modified for safety and comfort.
- Every yoga session should begin and end with several minutes of corpse pose (savasana) and quiet breathing.

Poses for the Spine

In combination, the following poses strengthen and stretch the back in the six natural directions of spinal movement (flexion, extension, lateral bending, and lateral twisting).

Seated Forward Fold: Pachimottanasana (pah-she-MOH-tahn-AHS-ahna)

In the seated position, extend your legs out in front of you, toes pointed up. Inhale, raising your arms above your head. Now exhale, reaching for your toes, ankles, or calves. Bending your knees if necessary, gently press the crown of your head towards your toes as you breathe deeply. Surrender to the breath.

Benefits	Contraindications
• Lengthens, tones, and flexes the spine	• Diarrhea
	• Pregnancy
	• Abdominal

- Relieves constipation and promotes digestion

- Regulates blood sugar levels

- Tones the kidneys

surgeries

Begin by lying on your stomach with your thighs parallel to each other. Firm your leg and thigh muscles as you extend your legs so that your toes push away from you towards the wall. As you inhale, place your elbows under your shoulders and your forearms on the floor. Exhale, using your chest muscles and back to lift your torso, without overextending, by pushing off with your hands.

Focus on rolling your outer thighs towards the floor, which lengthens your lower back and prevents it from being overly stressed. Stay in cobra for a few seconds, breathing deeply, and then slowly lower your chest to the floor. You can gradually increase to ten seconds. Turn your head to one side and take a few more breaths, feeling your back release and broaden. Repeat two to seven times.

Benefits	Contraindications
- Limbers the	- Hernia

- spine
- Strengthens muscles of the back, abdomen, and entire upper body
- Relieves gas and constipation
- Counteracts long hours sitting at a desk

- Peptic ulcers
- Pregnancy

Stand with your feet about three feet apart, turning your left foot slightly to the right and your right foot out to the right at 90 degrees. Raise your arms and reach them out to the sides, parallel to the floor, with the palms pointing down.

Anchor your left heel to the floor and firm your thighs, rolling your right thigh out. Breathe in, and as you exhale bend your right knee over the right ankle, so that the shin is perpendicular to the floor. Bend as far as is comfortable for you, bringing the right thigh as parallel to the floor as is right for your body. You can place your right hand along your calf or just outside your right foot, depending on your flexibility. You can also rest your right forearm on the top of the right thigh or place a block outside the front foot to support your hand.

Extend your left arm straight up toward the sky, and with a deep inhalation reach your left arm over the back of your left ear, with the palm facing down. Feel the stretch from your left heel through your left fingertips as you extend the entire left side of your body. Keep your gaze on your left hand (unless you have neck injuries) and focus on creating as much length on your right side as you have on the left side.

Hold the post for 10 to 30 seconds and come up on the inhale, pressing both heels into the floor, sweeping your left arm towards the sky. Reverse the position of your feet and repeat the sequence for the left side, holding the pose for the same length of time.

Benefits

Contraindications

- Strengthens and stretches the legs, knees, and ankles

- Promotes flexibility of the spine,

- Severe neck injuries

- Insomnia

- Headache

chest, groin, and
- shoulders
- Stimulates digestion

Sit on the floor with your legs out in front of you. Cross your bent left leg over your right thigh, placing your left foot on the floor. Place your right arm on the outside of your left knee and hold your right knee, while twisting your spine to the left. Hold this position, breathing easily. With every exhalation, allow yourself to surrender into the pose.

Return to the midline and repeat the posture on the other side by crossing your right leg over your left thigh, placing your right foot on the floor. Place your left arm on the outside of your right knee and hold your left knee, while twisting your spine to the right. Again, breathe easily into the pose, using your breath to increase your flexibility. As you become more flexible, reach around and grasp the ankle of the foot that is placed on the floor. Hold for ten seconds, then return to center.

Close your eyes for a few moments and put your attention on your spine. Envision the life force flowing up from the base of your spine, through your pelvis, into your abdomen, up through your heart, through your throat, between your eyes, and into your head. Imagine the thousand-petaled lotus flower at your crown chakra opening. Activate the intention to live your life from a more expanded state of awareness as a result of energy flowing freely through your body.

Benefits	Contraindications
*Lengthens the spine	• Herniated discs
• Massages and strengthens liver and kidneys	
• Stretches out chest and shoulder	

Poses for Knees and Hips

The following poses help stabilize the joints and strengthen the muscles around the knee and hip joints.

Triangle Pose: Trikonasana (trik-cone-AHS-ahna)

Bring your legs apart so your feet are wider than your shoulders. Raise both arms out to the side up to shoulder height so that they are parallel to the floor, palms turned down. Turn your left foot 90 degrees outward, keeping both hips facing forward. Turn your right foot slightly towards the left foot and keep the hips forward as if you have headlights coming from your hips, shining straight ahead.

Press your hips to the right and place your left hand on your thigh above your knee. Bring your right arm up so it is straight with fingertips toward the sky. Make sure to keep your body level as if you are between two glass window panes.

Hold pose for five or six breaths. Gradually return to an upright position, with your arms extended out to the sides, palms turned down. Pause for a moment. Repeat on the other side.

Modified Triangle: 5-Pointed Star

Stand with your legs apart. Keep both feet toes slightly turned out to side. Extend arms out to side. Take a breath in. When you exhale, place your left hand on the outside of your left thigh. The right arm extends up toward sky. Inhale, coming back to 5-pointed star, then exhale on the other side. Repeat 4 to 6 times.

Benefits	Contraindications
- Strengthens legs	- Knee injury
- Stretches inner thighs	- Neck injury
- Improves digestion and elimination	- Herniated disks
- Stimulates the abdominal organs	
- Helps relieve the symptoms	

of menopause

For most people the eagle pose is challenging on their first attempt; however, this pose can usually be mastered within a short period of time. It is helpful to do eagle arms and eagle legs separately for the first few times.

For most people the eagle pose is challenging on their first attempt; however, this pose can usually be mastered within a short period of time. It is helpful to do eagle arms and eagle legs separately for the first few times.

Arms

Extend your arms out to the side. Bend your left elbow in front of your body, fingertips up toward the sky and cross your right arm between your left arm and chest. Place the fingers of your right hand onto the palm of the left and point your fingertips to the ceiling. Gently press your elbows together. Hold this pose for ten seconds and then unwind.

Legs

Standing with your feet together, bend both knees, then shift your weight to your left foot. Raise your right leg, keeping both knees bent and then cross your right leg around the front of your left leg until you can hook your toes around your left calf muscle near the ankle. You will need to keep your left knee bent to achieve this. Repeat this balancing posture on the opposite side.

*When doing full Eagle, do the arms first and then follow instructions for legs.

Benefits

Contraindications

- Strengthens and stretches the ankles and calves

- Stretches the thighs, hips, shoulders & upper back

- Energizes and clears the lymph system

- Improves concentration

- Improves balance

- Knee injuries

- Ankle injuries

- Shoulder injuries

Stand with your legs three to four feet apart and turn your right foot in slightly to the right, and your left foot 90 degrees to the left. Align your left heel with your right heel. Expand your arms out stretching them parallel to the floor, with your palms facing down.

As you exhale, bend your left knee, bringing your left thigh as parallel to the floor as is comfortable for you. Keep expanding your arms away from your body keeping the torso long and the shoulders centered over your pelvis. Press your outer right heel into the floor and focus on firming the right leg as you bend the left knee. Don't allow your back to "sway" out; instead, keep the tailbone tilted slightly towards the pelvis. Stay in this position for five deep breaths. Come up on the inhale, reverse your feet, and repeat on the other side.

Benefits	Contraindications
- Strengthens the legs and knee muscles	- Knee injuries
- Stretches the shoulder and chest muscles	- Ankle injuries
- Increases groin flexibility	- Shoulder injuries
- Improves concentration	
- Improves balance	

- It's important not to hyperextend the knees in any pose, and be sure the knees and feet are in line. In standing poses, the feet should be firmly planted and toes spread apart.

- Some squatting, kneeling or one-legged poses may not be appropriate for certain people with arthritis in the knees, hips and ankles. Discuss this with your yoga instructor.

- If a muscle starts to feel fatigued, don't push it; just rest in corpse pose (savasana), lying comfortably on your back with your legs and arms slightly out.

- It is recommended that people with OA move through poses slowly, rather than holding one for a long period of time.

Ayurveda has many therapies to offer in the treatment of osteoarthritis. These include yoga, meditation, and the appropriate use of herbal therapies. These modalities offer their benefits without the significant risks associated with conventional medical treatments. By treating the underlying imbalances and by integrating body, mind, and spirit, we can develop a better connection to self and a better sense of health and happiness

Thanking You

Printed in Great
Britain
by Amazon